NATURAL WEIGHT LOSS

DR MIRIAM KINAI

ISBN: 1490575561

ISBN-13: 978-1490575568

CONTENTS

ACKNOWLEDGMENTS

I would like to express my sincere gratitude to everyone who contributed in one way or another to the development of this publication.

I would especially like to thank http://www.zazzle.com/ChristianArtGifts for their photographs.

1

DIET THERAPY

Dietary modifications that you can institute to lower your weight naturally include:

1.

Beans.

Eating beans, which are rich in fiber, helps reduce snacking between meals since one feels fuller longer. Beans also prevent the blood sugar surges and insulin spikes after meals that are associated with food cravings.

In addition, beans are said to increase levels of cholecystokinin which is a natural appetite suppressant.

Therefore, increase your intake of beans which are also good sources of protein, vitamins B1, B5, B9 and the antioxidant selenium.

***

2.

Eggs.

Eating eggs, especially for breakfast, helps reduce snacking during the day since they help a person feel fuller longer. Protein rich meals with eggs also prevent the blood sugar surges that are associated with food cravings.

In addition, eggs are also good sources of vitamin A, vitamin B12, the antioxidant selenium and useful amino acids like tryptophan and tyrosine.

Therefore eat poached or scrambled or boiled eggs for breakfast.

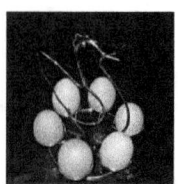

***

3.

Lentils.

Lentils are a good source of protein and thus reduce snacking by helping a person feel fuller for longer.

They are also high in fiber and this prevents the blood sugar surges that are associated with food cravings.

Lentils also contain resistant starch which is a type of carbohydrate that increases the body's metabolism and helps it burn more fat.

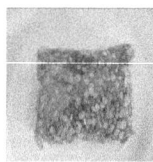

***

4.

Fish.

Fish contains an amino acid called leucine which can help a person lose weight while still maintaining their fat burning muscle.

Fish is also a good source of protein and this helps reduce snacking by making a person feel fuller longer and by preventing the blood sugar surges that are associated with food cravings.

Fish also contain vitamin B1, vitamin B3, vitamin B5, vitamin B6, vitamin B12 and the antioxidant selenium.

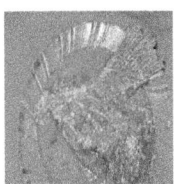

***

5.

Beef.

Lean beef contains an amino acid called leucine which can help a person lose weight while still maintaining their fat burning muscle.

Beef is also a good source of protein and this helps reduce snacking by making a person feel fuller longer and by preventing the blood sugar surges that are associated with food cravings.

In addition, beef is a good source of vitamin B1, vitamin B3, vitamin B5, vitamin B6, vitamin B9, vitamin B12 and the antioxidant selenium.

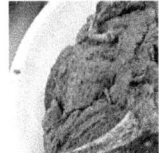

***

6.

Oats.

Oats are good sources of fiber which helps reduce snacking between meals by helping you feel fuller longer. Their high fiber content also prevents the blood sugar surges that are associated with food cravings.

In addition, oats boost the metabolism helping the body burn more fat.

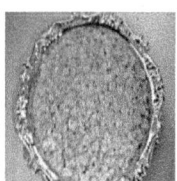

***

7.

High-Fiber Cereal.

Research has shown that eating high fiber cereals for breakfast can help a person eat less during the day by reducing their appetite.

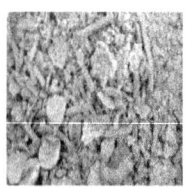

***

8.

Brown Rice.

Brown rice is a low calorie food that is also a good source of fiber and thus helps reduce snacking between meals by making a person feel fuller longer. It also boosts metabolism and helps the body burn fat.

***

9.

Nuts.

Snacking on a handful of nuts (150-160 calories) and especially almonds has been shown to result in weight loss. This is because nuts are filling and thus result in less food consumption at the subsequent meals.

In addition, eating nuts also boosts the metabolism and thus helps the body burn more fat.

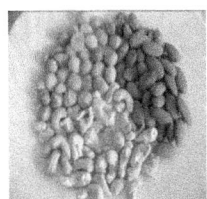

***

10.

Broccoli.

Increase your intake of raw or cooked broccoli since it is low in calories and has a high in fiber content which helps reduce snacking between meals.

In addition, it also contains cancer-preventing nutrients, omega 3 fatty acids, vitamin B3, vitamin B5, vitamin C and iron.

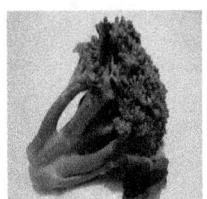

***

11.

Grapefruit.

Research has shown that eating half a grapefruit before meals or drinking one serving of its juice three times a day can help a person lose weight or up to one pound each week.

Grapefruits also contain a chemical that can reduce insulin levels and consequently fat storage.

In addition, they are a low calorie food since one grapefruit contains around 100 calories.

***

12.

Pears.

Pears are rich in pectin fiber which helps reduce snacking between meal by lowering blood glucose levels and helping you feel fuller longer.

Their fiber content is also quite high since one pear provides 15% of the daily recommended intake. This high fiber content helps prevents the blood sugar surges that are associated with food cravings.

Therefore eat three pears each day with their skins since the fiber is in the skin.

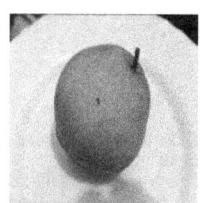

***

13.

Blueberries.

Blueberries are rich in fiber which helps reduce snacking between meals by helping you feel fuller longer.

Their high fiber content also prevents the blood sugar surges that are associated with food cravings.

Black berries are also low in calories since one cup of blueberries provides less than 100 calories.

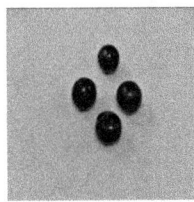

***

14.

Apples.

Apples are rich in pectin fiber which helps reduce snacking between meal by lowering blood glucose levels and helping you feel fuller longer.

Their high fiber content also prevents the blood sugar surges that are associated with food cravings.

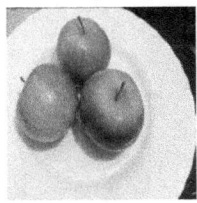

***

15.

Bananas.

Bananas contain resistant starch which helps the body's metabolism increase and thus it is able to burn more fat. Slightly green bananas provide more resistant starch than ripe ones.

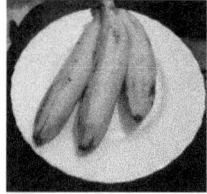

***

16.

Oranges.

Oranges perfect weight loss foods since they are low in calories at around 50 each and high fiber and water content.

They therefore help a person feel full for longer and thus they are less likely to eat between meals.

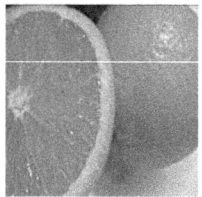

***

17.

Green tea.

Research has shown that drinking 5 cups of green tea each day can help a person lose weight. This is due to the fact it contains chemicals known as catechins which can boost the metabolism and increase the body's fat burning ability.

Green tea also contains antioxidants which protect the body from free radical damage and lower levels of the bad LDL cholesterol. It is also filling since it mainly water. Therefore drink green tea each day.

***

18.

Milk.

Milk contains fatty acids that help a person feel full longer and therefore less likely to snack. They also help the body burn more fat.

In addition, upping your daily milk intake to ensure that you consume 1000 to 1400 milligrams of calcium has been shown by studies to increase the amount of fat and calories that the body burns.

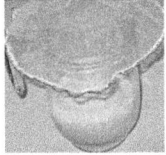

***

19.

Cheese.

Feta and goat cheese from grass fed animals contains fatty acids that help a person feel full longer and therefore less likely to snack. They also help the body burn more fat.

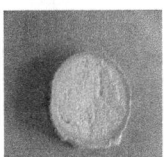

***

20.

Tofu.

Eating tofu as a snack or an appetizer has been shown to be so filling that it can lead to less food consumption during the subsequent meal.

21.

Olive Oil.

Olive oil is one of those monounsaturated fat that can help a person burn fat since they boost metabolism.

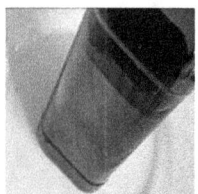

22.

Vinegar.

Eating bread that has been dipped in vinegar has been shown to help people feel fuller longer.

* * * * *

2

SUPPLEMENTS

Nutritional supplements that can help lower weight naturally include:

1.

Hoodia

Hoodia Gordonii is obtained from a plant that grows in the Kalahari Desert in South Africa. It is used for weight loss because it is believed to be an appetite suppressant that increases feelings of fullness. This helps decrease calorie consumption without feelings of deprivation.

2.

Chitosan

Chitosan is obtained from lobsters, crab and shrimp. It is used for weight loss because it reduces the absorption of fats.

3.

Green Tea Extract

Green tea extract is used for weight loss because it is believed to reduce the appetite and boost fat metabolism. It has also been found to help obese persons reduce their BMI.

***

4.

Fiber

If you are not able to get adequate fiber from your diet, consider taking a fiber supplement since this will help you fell fuller for longer. As you do so, ensure that you increase your water intake to avoid constipation.

***

5.

Chromiun Picolate

Chromiun picolate reduces sugar cravings by stabilizing the metabolism of simple carbohydrates.

***

6.

Calcium

Calcium is involved in the metabolism of lipase which is an enzyme that is involved in fat digestion. Women on a diet who took 1000 mg of calcium each day were found to have lost more weight and body fat than those who were given a placebo though the differences were not statistically significant. Therefore increase your intake of low fat dairy foods.

***

7.

Daily Multivitamin

A multi-vitamin and multi-mineral supplement that is well balanced and that contains the nutrients in their daily recommended values should be taken every day.

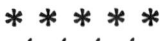

3

HERBS

Herbs that are used for weight loss include:

1.

Cayenne Pepper

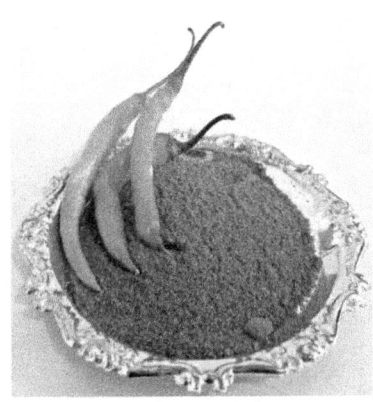

Cayenne pepper contains a compound known as capsaicin which is useful for managing weight because it helps reduce caloric intake. It also increases the process of thermogenesis in the body in which fat is burnt to produce heat. Thermogenesis increases the metabolic rate of the body enabling it to burn more calories.

***

2.

Black Pepper

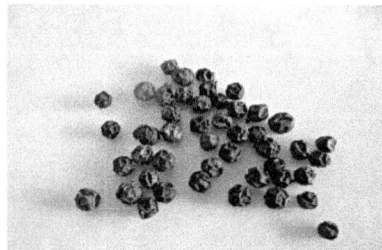

Black pepper contains a compound known as piperine which reduces the formation of fat cells. It also increases metabolism and helps the body burn more calories especially when it is combined with thermogenic foods like cayenne pepper.

***

3.

Ginger

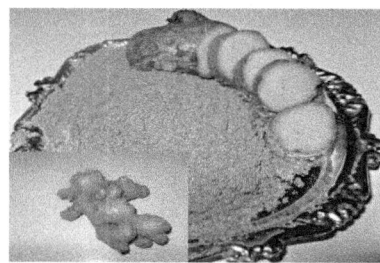

Ginger is used for weight loss because it increase thermogenesis. This is the process by which the body produces heat and in so doing burns calories. Ginger is also said to act as an appetite suppressant by increasing satiety and thus it can help reduce caloric intake.

***

4.

Turmeric

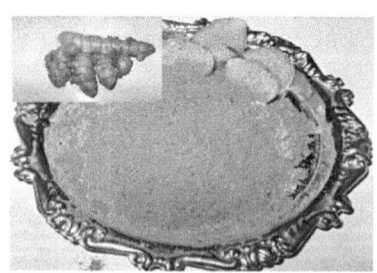

Turmeric contains curcumin which is thought to reduce adipose (fat) tissue formation.

***

5.

Cinnamon

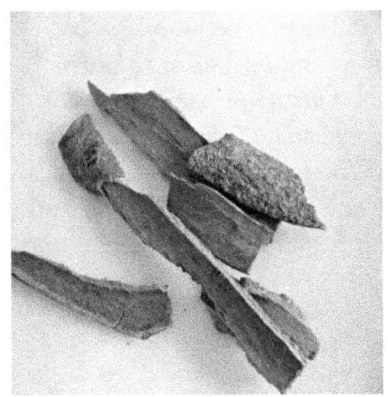

Cinnamon is used for weight loss since it is thought to increase the body's metabolism thereby enabling it to burn more fat. Cinnamon also helps regulate blood glucose levels by reducing the insulin surges that occur after meals and contribute to food cravings. It is therefore doubly effective for diabetics trying to lose weight.

In addition, persons with type 2 diabetes who take one quarter of a teaspoon of cinnamon each day are able to reduce their blood glucose, cholesterol and triglyceride levels.

***

6.

Mustard

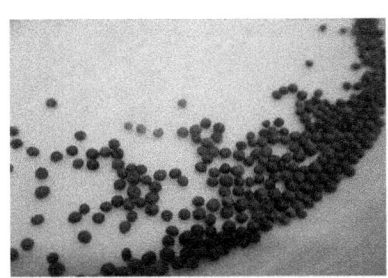

Mustard seeds increase the body's metabolism helping it burn more calories. Therefore consider adding half a teaspoon of mustard seeds to your diet each day since this can help you burn more calories even when you are resting.

***

7.

Cardamom

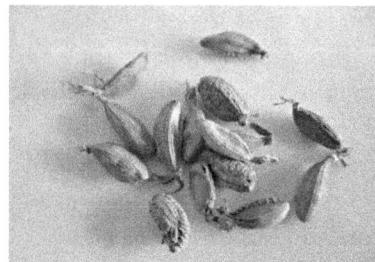

Cardamon boosts the body's metabolism and enables it to burn more fat by virtue of being a thermogenic spice. This means that it increases the process of thermogenesis in which the body produces heat and burns calories in the process of doing so.

***

8.

Cumin

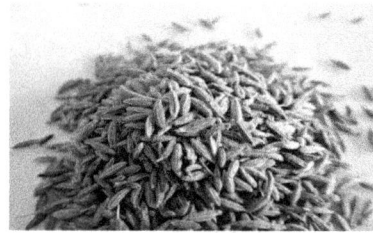

Cumin is used for weight loss since it aids the production of energy by the body.

***

9.

Guar

Guar which is also known as guar gum and jaguar gum is obtained from the Indian cluster plant seed. It is used for weight loss because it is believed to reduce fat absorption. It also helps a person feel fuller for longer and this can contribute to decreased calorie consumption.

Avoid guar if you have diabetes since it can cause fluctuations in the blood sugar levels. Guar can also cause intestinal obstruction since it can swell up to 20 times its original size.

***

10.

Dandelion

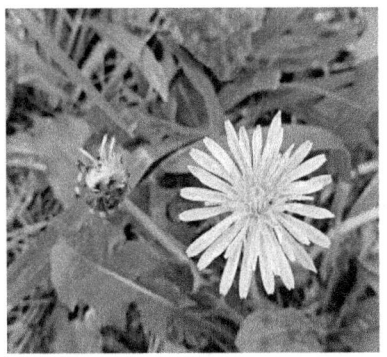

Dandelions are useful for weight loss because they are rich in fiber and make a person feel fuller for longer. They are thus able to reduce snacking between meals. Dandelions are also natural diuretics. This means they make a person pass urine more frequently and this may also contribute to weight loss.

Avoid dandelion if you are allergic to aster family plants like daisies, ragweed, marigolds and chrysanthemums.

***

11.

Garcinia Cambodge

Garcinia is believed to be an appetite suppressant even though it is not a stimulant.

If you have diabetes or alzheimers do not take garcinia since it can upset blood glucose regulation.

***

12.

Siberian Ginseng

Siberian ginseng (Eleutherococcus senticosus) is used for weight loss because it is believed to increase energy levels and boost the body's metabolism. This helps the body burn more fat even when it is resting. It is also thought to help the body adjust to a new weight loss program.

* * * * *
, , , ,

4

ESSENTIAL OILS

Aromatherapy oils that are used for weight loss include:

The top notes:

Grapefruit essential oil

Lemon essential oil

The middle notes:

Peppermint essential oil

The base notes:

Sandalwood essential oil

Patchouli essential oil

***

Grapefruit Essential Oil

Botanical Name: Citrus paradisi

Method of Extraction: Cold pressed from fruit peel

Perfumery Note: Top note

Aromatic Description: Refreshing, tangy sweet and citrusy

**

Grapefruit Essential Oil Safety Information

1. Do not expose skin to the sun or UV rays for 24 hours after using it.

***

Lemon Essential Oil

Botanical Name: Citrus limon

Method of Extraction: Expressed

Perfumery Note: Top note

Aromatic Description: Fresh citrus

**

Lemon Essential Oil Safety Information

1. Do not use it if skin will be exposed to sunlight or UV rays in 12-24 hours as it is phototoxic.

2. Do not use it if you have low blood pressure.

3. It may irritate sensitive skin.

4. Do not use it if you are allergic to lemons.

***

Peppermint Essential Oil

Botanical Name: Mentha piperita

Method of Extraction: Steam distilled

Perfumery Note: Middle note

Odor Intensity: 7

Strength of Initial Aroma: Strong

Aromatic Description: Minty

**

Peppermint Essential Oil Safety Information

1. Do not use it in pregnancy.

2. Do not use it if you are breastfeeding.

3. Do not use it on children less than 5 years.

4. Do not use it if you have epilepsy.

5. Do not use it if you have irregular heart beats or cardiac fibrillation.

6. Avoid it if you have high blood pressure.

7. Do not use it before using a sun bed or going to hot humid places.

8. Do not store it near homeopathic products as it may affect them.

9. It may cause sleeplessness if used in the night.

10. Do not use on damaged or sensitive skin.

***

Sandalwood Essential Oil

Botanical Name: Santalum album

Method of Extraction: Steam distilled

Perfumery Note: Base note

Odor Intensity: 5

Strength of Initial Aroma: Medium

Aromatic Description: Sweet, woody

**

Sandalwood Essential Oil Safety Information

1. Avoid using sandalwood if you are allergic to balsams.

2. Do not use it alone for more than 2-3 months as it may lead to sensitization.

3. Always buy your essential oils from a reputable vender to ensure you use high quality therapeutic grade essential oils in your blends.

4. Do not confuse essential oils with fragrance oils as the latter are not the natural essences.

***

Patchouli Essential Oil

Botanical Name: Pogostemon cablin

Method of Extraction: Steam distilled

Color: Dark yellow brown

Perfumery Note: Base note

Odor Intensity:

Strength of Initial Aroma: Medium

Aromatic Description: Musky and spicy

**

Patchouli Essential Oil Safety Information

1. If used in large amounts may cause anorexia or loss of appetite in some people.

2. Do not use/ avoid it if you are allergic to cosmetics, perfumes and spicy foods

3. Always buy your essential oils from a reputable vender to ensure you use high quality therapeutic grade essential oils in your blends.

4. Do not confuse essential oils with fragrance oils as the latter are not the natural essences.

***

Natural Weight Loss Essential Oil Recipes

The first step in using essential oils is to do a patch test on each of the essential oils that you want to use.

To do this, simply apply the essential oil that has been diluted with a carrier oil on the inner aspect of your elbow, bandage it and wait for 24 hours to see if you will develop rashes or itchiness or swelling or any other sign of an allergic reaction. If you do, do not use that essential oil.

The second step is to create the essential oil blend that you will use to help you lose weight. A simple "Weight Loss Blend" can be made by mixing 10 drops of sandalwood essential oil, 20 drops of peppermint essential oil and 30 drops of lemon essential oil.

We will refer to this mixture as the "Weight Loss Blend" in our recipes. Therefore, if the recipe says, "Add 12 drops of the Weight Loss Blend", simply add 12 drops of this mixture of essential oils.

If you only want to experiment with one essential oil, I would recommend lemon essential oil.

***

Scent Balls.

Add 6 drops of lemon essential oil or 6 drops of the "Weight Loss Blend" to a handkerchief or a cotton ball and sniff it before your meals. Ensure that you sniff it at least 3 times each day. You can also sniff it before your exercise sessions to help you feel more energized.

If you want to manage the stress and anxiety that make you overeat, inhale lavender essential oil. If you want to manage the sadness and depression that make you overeat, inhale rosemary essential oil.

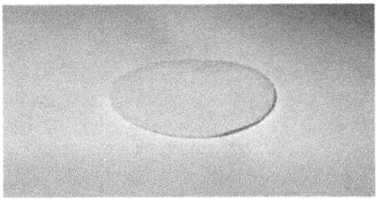

Scented Salts.

Mix 1 cup Epsom salts with 1 cup sea salt and add 50 drops (2.5 ml) of lemon essential oil or 6 drops of the "Weight Loss Blend" in a glass jar with a tight lid. Open the jar and take a whiff of the scent whenever you need to fight a craving.

If you want to manage the stress and anxiety that make you overeat, add 50 drops of lavender essential oil. If you want to manage the sadness and depression that make you overeat, add 50 drops of rosemary essential oil.

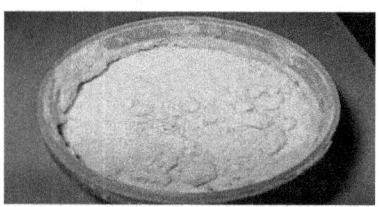

Personal perfume.

Put 10 ml jojoba in a spray bottle and add 50 drops of the "Weight Loss Blend" followed by 10 ml of 99% alcohol isopropyl to make your own perfume. Let your perfume stand for at least 2 days or for even up to 6 weeks because the longer it stands, the stronger it will be.

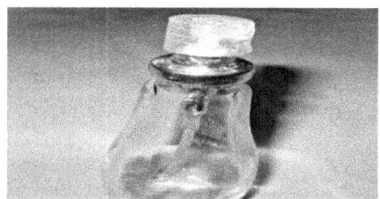

Body Splash.

Add 50 drops of the "Weight Loss Blend" to one cup (8 oz or 250 ml) of distilled water in a spray bottle and use it to spray your body whenever you need to overcome a craving.

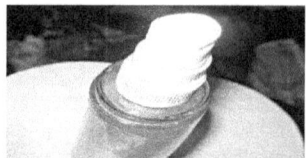

Room Fragrance.

Add 24 drops of the "Weight Loss Blend" to your diffuser. If your diffuser comes with instructions, use the number of drops recommended by the manufacturer.

If you want to manage the stress and anxiety that make you overeat, use lavender essential oil.

If you want to manage the sadness and depression that make you overeat, use rosemary essential oil.

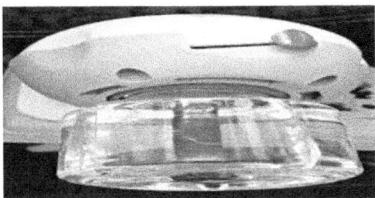

Room Scent.

Add 12 drops of the "Weight Loss Blend" to ¼ cup (2 oz or 60 ml) of water, place it on an oil warmer and light the candle to scatter the "anti-smoking" scent in the room.

If you want to manage the stress and anxiety that make you overeat, use lavender essential oil.

If you want to manage the sadness and depression that make you overeat, use rosemary essential oil.

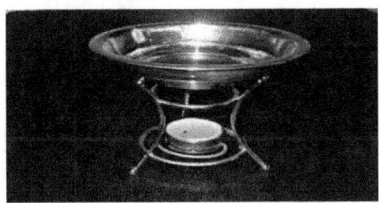

Car Diffuser.

Add the "Weight Loss Blend" to your car's diffuser according to the manufacturer's instructions and let the "anti-smoking" scent envelope you as you drive.

If you want to manage the stress and anxiety that make you overeat, use lavender essential oil. If you want to manage the sadness and depression that make you overeat, use rosemary essential oil.

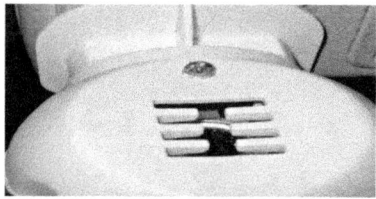

Air Freshener.

Create your own air freshener by adding 250 drops (12.5 ml or 2.5 teaspoons) of the "Weight Loss Blend" to one cup (8 oz or 250 ml) of water in a spray bottle and spray it around your room.

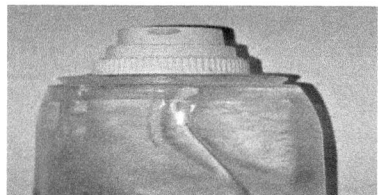

Potpourri.

Add 250 drops of the "Weight Loss Blend" to one cup of dried roses, lavender buds, cloves and cinnamon sticks. Mix thoroughly and put the mixture in a lid with a tight jar. Let it stand for 1 week as you continue shaking the bottle without opening it.

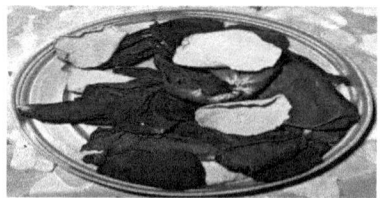

Body Massage Oil.

Add 50 drops of the "Weight Loss Blend" to one cup (8 oz or 250 ml) of sweet almond oil or any other carrier oil to create a healing body massage oil. Get a professional massage or do a self massage paying special attention to the thighs and hips.

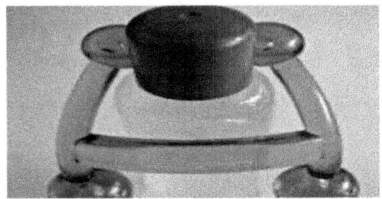

Mini Self Massage Oil.

Add 3 drops of the "Weight Loss Blend" to 10 ml of sweet almond oil or any other carrier oil and put it in a small bottle that can fit into your purse or pocket. Carry it with you for 5 minute mini – self massages for your temples or the back of your neck whenever you feel the urge to eat between your meals.

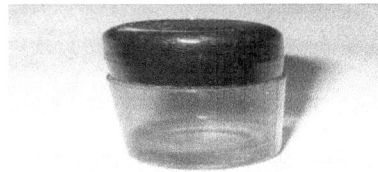

Body Dry Brushing.

Add 2 drops of the "Weight Loss Blend" to the natural bristles of a bath brush and brush your entire skin before bathing to stimulate it and get rid of the dead skin cells. Dry brushing is also thought to help break up the cellulite. Start from your feet and work your way up the heart.

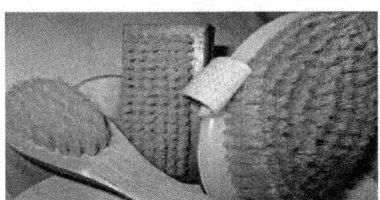

Aromatherapy Bath.

Create weight loss bath by dispersing 20 drops of the "Weight Loss Blend" in warm bath water. Mix it with milk to help it disperse.

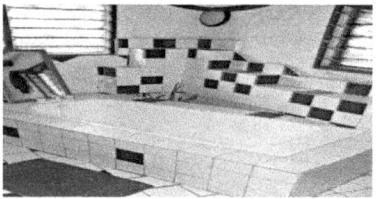

Bath Gel.

Add 50 drops of the "Weight Loss Blend" to one cup (8 oz or 250 ml) of an unscented liquid soap to create an Weight Loss bath gel.

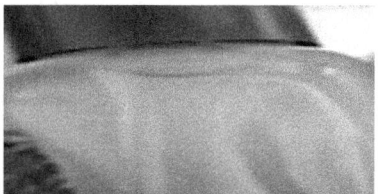

Bath Gloves and Bath Mitts Massage

Pour the aromatherapy bath gel on bath gloves or bath mitts. Using circular movements, massage your body from the feet to the heart.

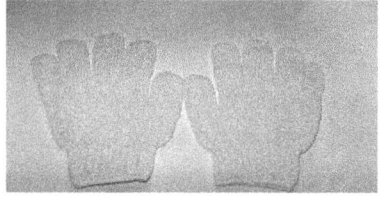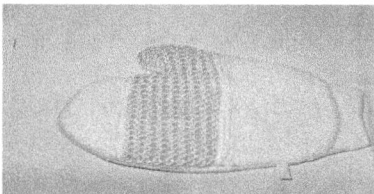

Bath Salts.

Mix 2 cups Epsom salts, 1 cup sea salt and 1 cup baking soda. Add 50 drops of the "Weight Loss Blend" and a few drops of food coloring (optional). Add one cup of these bath salts to your warm bath water.

Bath Tea.

Mix 2 cups of herbs like lavender flowers, dried lemon rind and rosemary leaves with 25 drops of the "Weight Loss Blend" and 1 cup of sea salt. Put the mixture in an air tight jar or you can add a scoopful of the mixture into a cotton bath tea bag and store the filled bath tea bags in the air tight jar.

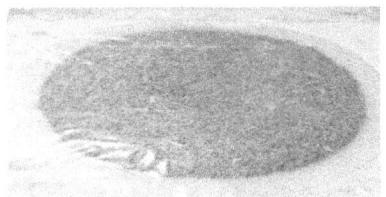

Body Scrub.

Scrub the stress away by adding 50 drops of the "Weight Loss Blend" to one cup (8 oz or 250 ml) of sweet almond oil or any other carrier oil. Mix it with ½ cup of Epsom salts or brown sugar or white sugar. Rub if all over your body to remove the dead skin cells then rinse it off to reveal baby soft skin.

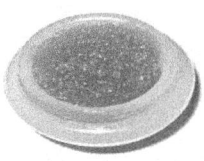

Body Oil.

Add 50 drops of the "Weight Loss Blend" to one cup (8 oz or 250 ml) of sweet almond oil or sunflower oil or any other carrier oil and use it as an after shower body oil. Massage it into your skin after patting it dry, but while it is still moist.

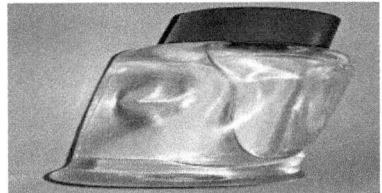

Handy Massager.

Apply the Weight Loss massage oil and use the handy massager to give yourself a self-massage.

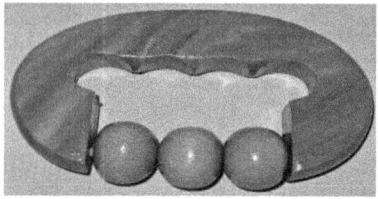

Body Lotion.

Heat 6 oz (190 ml) of sweet almond oil and 1.5 oz (45 grams) of grated beeswax in a double boiler until they mix. Remove from the heat and let the mixture cool completely. Put 8 oz (250 ml) water in a blender and with the blender on high speed, slowly pour in the cooled vegetable oil and beeswax mixture. Blend until the mixture emulsifies or forms a thick lotion. Add 15 drops of the "Weight Loss Blend" to. Pour the lotion in a glass jar.

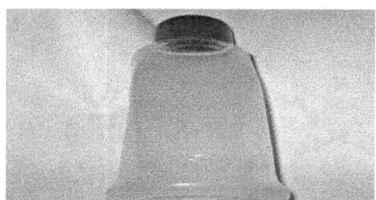

Aloe Vera Aromatherapy Gel.

Add 50 drops of the "Weight Loss Blend" to one cup (8 oz or 250 ml) of natural aloe vera gel to create a non-greasy, healing moisturizer.

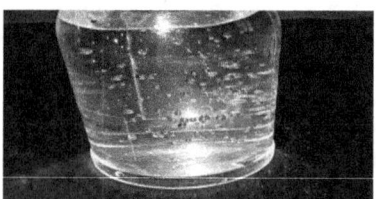

Foot Bath.

Create your own healing foot bath blend by adding 50 drops of the "Weight Loss Blend" to a bowl of warm water to soak your feet.

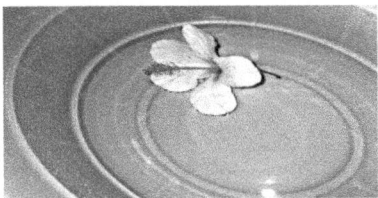

Foot Oil.

Add 25 drops of the "Weight Loss Blend" to ½ cup (4 oz or 125 ml) ml of virgin coconut oil or any other carrier oil. Use it to massage your feet after the foot bath and before you wrap them in soft cotton socks.

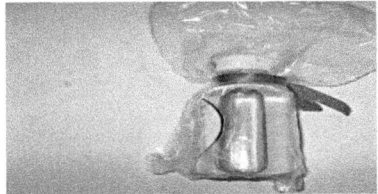

Healing Salve.

Melt 1 oz. (30 grams) of beeswax with 8 oz. (250 ml or 1 cup) of olive oil or any other vegetable oil in a double boiler. Remove from the heat source and one the mixture cools add up to 50 drops (2.5 ml or ½ teaspoon) of the "Weight Loss Blend" to drop by drop until you get your preferred scent. Pour the mixture into storage tins and allow it to cool completely.

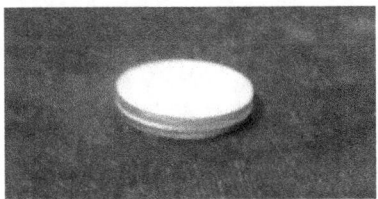

Beeswax Cream.

Melt 4 tablespoons of beeswax and 2 tablespoons of shea butter. Remove from the heat source and add 8 tablespoons of sweet almond oil or any other carrier oil you may have. Mix thoroughly and when the mixture cools, add 12 drops of the "Weight Loss Blend".

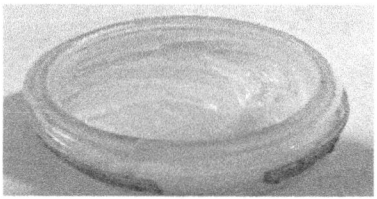

Petroleum Jelly Hand Cream.

Melt 2 teaspoons of a petroleum jelly like Vaseline, add 6 drops of the "Weight Loss Blend" to when cool and then pour into a jar.

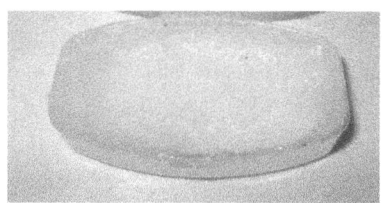

* * * * *

5

LIFESTYLE MODIFICATIONS

Lifestyle modifications that can help you lose weight naturally include:

1.

Regular Exercise

Regular exercise is very important for weight loss since the body burns calories during the exercise sessions. Weight bearing exercises help increase muscle mass which helps the body burn more calories even when it is resting.

***

2.

Stress Management

Emotional stress can make a person increase their intake of comfort foods like cakes and mashed potatoes.

Therefore learn and practice relaxation techniques so that you can manage stress effectively to stop emotional eating.

3.

Get Adequate Sleep

Get 7-10 hours of sleep every night since it can help you maintain a normal body weight. This is due to the fact that the production of grehlin, an appetite stimulant, by the body decreases during sleep while that of letpin, an appetite suppressant, increases.

4.

Limit Alcohol Intake

Reduce your alcohol intake since it is full of empty calories and drinking can also lead to mindless excessive consumption of calorie dense foods.

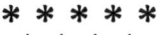

7

WEIGHT LOSS PLAN

Before you embark on a weight loss plan, consult your doctor and nutritionist since your medications and diet may need to be tweaked.

Once you have been medically and nutritionally cleared, follow the steps in our healthy weight loss plan which involves loosing 1 pound or 500 grams or ½ kg of body fat each week.

To lose 1 pound of fat each week you have to cut 500 calories from your diet each day or burn 500 calories each day.

Know Your Lifestyle

The first step of this plan is to calculate the number of calories you need to eat to maintain your current weight. This number is determined by whether you live a sedentary or active lifestyle:

Sedentary Lifestyle

Characteristics of a sedentary lifestyle include:

a. At work you sit at a desk all day typing or reading (e.g. accountant, lawyer, blogger) or you are seated driving (delivery service, cab driver)

b. At home you spend most of your time seated working on the computer or watching TV

c. You rarely or never exercise

If you lead a sedentary lifestyle, the number of calories you need to eat to maintain your current weight is Your weight in pounds X 13 or Your weight in kilograms X 26.

To lose weight healthily, you need to cut out 500 calories from this number each day.

For example if you weigh 200 pounds or 100 kg, you need to eat (200 lb X 13 = 2600 calories) or (100 kg X 26 = 2600 calories) each day to maintain your body weight.

To lose weight healthily, you need to eat 2600 - 500 = 2100 calories each day if you weigh 200 pounds or 100 kg and lead a sedentary lifestyle.

Light Activity Lifestyle

Characteristics of a light activity lifestyle include:

a. At work you walk around for more than 2 hours each day (e.g. waitress, teacher, nurse)

b. At home you walk around a lot doing light housework (e.g. ironing, dusting, making beds, hanging the washing) and light gardening (e.g. raking leaves).

c. You exercise by taking long leisurely walks or workout in a gym for less than 2 hours each week in a gym or at home

If you lead a light activity lifestyle, the number of calories you need to eat to maintain your current weight is Your weight in pounds X 14 or Your weight in kilograms X 28.

To lose weight healthily, you need to cut out 500 calories from this number each day.

Moderate Activity Lifestyle

Characteristics of a moderate activity lifestyle include:

a. At work you run around all day (e.g. errand boy) or do physically demanding jobs (e.g. carpenter, mechanic)

b. At home you do rarely sit as you do heavy housework and gardening (e.g. pushing power mower)

c. You exercise by brisk walking, dancing or working out for a total of 3 to 5 hours each week in a gym or at home

If you lead a moderate activity lifestyle, the number of calories you need to eat to maintain your current weight is Your weight in pounds X 15 or Your weight in kilograms X 30.

To lose weight healthily, you need to cut out 500 calories from this number each day.

Active Lifestyle

Characteristics of an active lifestyle include:

a. At work you do heavy manual labor (e.g. construction site job)

b. At home you spend most of your time physically active (e.g. pushing hand mower, chopping wood, home repairs and renovation)

c. You exercise for several hours each day in a gym or at home or engage in physical sport such as playing lawn tennis, jogging or mountain biking each day.

If you lead an active lifestyle, the number of calories you need to eat to maintain your current weight is Your weight in pounds X 16 or Your weight in kilograms X 32.

To lose weight healthily, you need to cut out 500 calories from this number each day.

Therefore, use your current weight and activity level to calculate the number of calories you need to eat each day to lose weight healthily.

Cut Out 500 Calories

To lose weight healthily by shedding 1 pound or 500 gm or ½ kg of body fat each week, you need to cut out 500 calories from your diet each day. Therefore, go through the following food calories list to see the foods you can omit each day to cut out 500 calories from your eating plan.

Approximately 500 Calorie Meals

3 medium plain baked potatoes or 5 medium boiled potatoes or 5 medium five inch sweet potatoes

3-egg omelette with cheese or 4 large egg omelettes or 5 boiled eggs

3 medium portions boiled rice or boiled spaghetti

180 grams bran flakes or 10 Weetabix biscuits

1 bacon beefburger or cheeseburger

10 bacon rasher of 25 grams

5 slices bread or 3 chapatis

300 grams grilled chicken

6 fried chicken wings

1 serving chips

4 beef sausages

Approximately 500 Calorie Vegetables

60 cups shredded lettuce or 20 cups green beans or 20 cups spinach

10 medium portion boileds peas or 2 medium cabbages boiled

20 bell peppers or 20 seven-inch carrots or 20 tomatoes

10 cucumbers or 10 medium stalk broccoli

4 cauliflowers

Approximately 500 Calorie Fruits

5 medium apples or 5 medium bananas or 5 medium grapefruits or 5 pears or 5 mangoes

10 medium oranges or 10 tangerines or 50 lemons

10 cups diced watermelon or 5 cups grapes

100 strawberries or 10 dried figs

2 medium avocados

20 slices pineapples

Approximately 500 Calorie Snacks

1 cup raisins or 1 cup mixed nuts

100 roasted peanuts

36 macadamia nuts

15 cups popcorn

Approximately 500 Calorie Desserts

6 level tablespoons peanut butter or 10 teaspoons honey or 5 tablespoons mayonnaise

3 slices fruitcake or 2 pieces iced, chocolate double layer cake

5 biscuits or 5 cookies or 3 doughnuts

100 gram dairy milk chocolate

10 teaspoons sugar

Approximately 500 Calorie Drinks

500 ml or 1 pint skimmed milk

5 medium portions porridge

600 ml drinking chocolate

20 mugs unsweetened tea

5 cups vegetable soup

3 pints (1500 ml) beer

5 cups low fat milk

3 bottles soft drink

600 ml red wine

***

Burn 500 Calories

To lose weight healthily by shedding 1 pound or 500 gm or ½ kg of body fat each week you can also burn 500 calories each day. Therefore, choose from the following list the activities you can engage in to burn 500 calories each day.

To burn approximately 500 calories, you can do the following activities for 30 minutes:

Rollerblading, running at 8 mph

To burn approximately 500 calories, you can do the following activities for 45 minutes:

Jumping a rope, running at 6.5 mph

To burn approximately 500 calories, you can do the following activities for 1 hour:

Rock climbing, jogging at 5 mph, swimming, backpacking, mountain biking, cross country skiing, running up stairs, walking fast uphill, spinning class, high impact aerobics, playing tennis, playing squash or racquetball, playing basketball, playing football, playing volleyball.

To burn approximately 500 calories, you can do the following activities for 1 hour and 15 minutes:

Hiking, playing golf while carrying your clubs, surfing, pushing a lawn mower, gardening, heavy housework, walking up stairs, dancing, washing the car, aerobics class.

To burn approximately 500 calories, you can do the following activities for 2 hours and 30 minutes:

Taking a walk at 3 mph, Playing badminton, walking at a leisurely pace, cooking, rowing a boat at a leisurely pace.

* * * * *

7

EXERCISE PLAN

A balanced exercise plan should combine stretching, weight bearing and aerobic exercises.

If you have been leading a sedentary lifestyle, consult your doctor and nutritionist before making changes to your exercise regimen.

In addition, invest in a good pair of sports shoes that will cushion your feet and redistribute your weight evenly as you walk, jog, jump or run.

If as you exercise, you experience any of the following symptoms, stop exercising at once and consult your doctor: chest pain, pressure or tightness, unusual shortness of breath, pain in the jaw, arm, neck or shoulder, palpitations or skipped heart beats, feeling dizzy or fainting, muscle pain that is more severe than just discomfort.

1.

Stretching Exercises

Stretch for at least 10 minutes each morning and evening and in the warm up and cool down periods just before or right after your exercise sessions.

To stretch correctly you should:

1. Not hold your breath as you stretch. Breathe in and out rhythmically.

2. Never bounce into or out of your stretches. Gently move into and out of the various positions.

3. Hold the stretch position for 10 seconds and gradually increase the duration.

4. Be systematic and begin with the legs as you work your way up the body to the neck or vice versa.

5. Stop stretching if you feel any pain but continue if you experience mild discomfort.

The following is a list of exercises that you can do at home to stretch your entire body.

1. Neck Stretch - Stand with your feet shoulder width apart and your chin on your chest. Rotate your head once clockwise. Return chest to chin and rotate it counter clockwise. Do several rotations. Turn your face to the right, look as far back over your shoulder as you can. Hold for a count of 10. Repeat on opposite side.

2. Chest, Shoulder and Arm Stretch - Stand with your feet shoulder width apart and your knees slightly bent. Clasp your hands behind your back and push them back as far as you can reach. Push your chest forward as far as it can reach. Hold and return to starting position.

3. Side Stretch - Stand straight with your arms raised over your head. Tilt your body to the left side as you stretch your side muscles. Hold. Repeat on the opposite side.

4. Abs, Glutes and Quads Stretch - Stand with your feet together. Reach forward with your right arm. Lift your left leg behind you and grasp your left ankle with your left hand. Lift your left thigh as high as you can or until it is parallel to the ground. Repeat on opposite side.

5. Back Stretch - Lie on your back and pull both knees to your chest. Release them and lower your knees to the right side and then to the left side. Return knees back to chest.

6. Hamstring Stretch - Lie on your back with your legs bent and both feet flat on the floor. Straighten and raise your right leg. Gently pull your right thigh towards your body and hold for a count of 10. Repeat on the opposite side.

***

2.

Weight Bearing Exercises

To weight train or strength train correctly you should:

a) Not hold your breath or strain as you train.

b) Not exercise the same muscle groups for two consecutive days.

c) Aim for 3 sets of 10 repetitions each.

The following are exercises that you can do at home to strength train your entire body.

1. Overhead Press - (Works shoulders) Sit on a chair; hold a weight (or a full water bottle) in each hand at shoulder level with palms facing forward. Raise your arms straight up over your head. Lower them to shoulder level.

2. Biceps Curl - (Works biceps) Sit on a chair; hold a weight (or a full water bottle) in each hand palms facing forward. Bend your elbow and lift the weight towards your shoulder. Return to starting position and repeat with the other arm.

3. Triceps Dips - (Works triceps) Sit on the edge of a sturdy chair with your back and shoulders straight. Hold the edge of a chair and bend your elbows to form a right angle as you lower your butt off the seat to the floor. Straighten your arms and press back up to raise your butt back to the seat.

4. Push Ups - (Works deltoids, triceps, pectorals) Lie on floor, palms face down, elbows bent next to shoulders. Push up from floor by straightening elbows and contracting abs so that your body forms a straight line from your head to heel (beginners can rest both knees on floor) Lower yourself to floor by bending elbows. Push back up.

5. Simple Straight Crunches - (Works abs) Lie flat on your back; bend knees while keeping your feet flat on the floor. Place your hands on your thighs. Exhale and lift shoulder blades from the floor as you slide your hands up to your knees. Hold for a count of 10. Return to starting position and repeat.

6. Simple Side Crunches - (Works abs) Lie flat on your back; bend knees while keeping your feet flat on the floor. Place your hands on your right thigh. Exhale and lift shoulder blades from the floor as you slide your hands up to your right knee. Hold for a count of 10. Return to starting position and repeat. Do on opposite side.

7. Advanced Straight Crunches - (Works abs) Lie flat on your back; bend your knees until thighs are perpendicular to floor. Place arms crossed over your chest. Exhale, tighten abs and lift shoulder blades from the floor as you reach towards knees. Hold for a count of 10. Return to starting position and repeat.

8. Advanced Side Crunches - (Works abs) Lie flat on your back; bend your knees until thighs are perpendicular to floor. Place arms crossed over your chest. Exhale, tighten abs and lift shoulder blades from floor as you reach towards right knee. Hold for a count of 10. Return to starting position and repeat. Do on opposite side.

9. Leg Lifts - Lie on your back; legs straight; hands under butt. Lift legs 30 cm from the floor. Hold for a count of 10.

10. Lunge - (Works glutes, hamstrings, quadriceps) Stand with feet shoulder width apart, arms at sides. Take a large step forward with your left leg and ensure your left knee is above your left foot. Lower your body to the floor by bending the right knee until right thigh is parallel to the floor and right knee is close to the ground. Squeeze your glutes as you press back up to your starting position. Repeat on opposite side.

11. Squat - (Works your butt and thighs) Stand with your feet parallel and shoulder width apart. Stretch out your hands in front of you. Keeping your abs and butt tight, bend your knees and slowly lower yourself as though you are sitting. Ensure your knees don't extend past your toes. Hold for a count of 10. As your rise, squeeze your glutes.

12. Calf Raises - (Work your calf muscles) Stand with feet together and arms raised above your head. Lift your heels so that you are standing on the balls of your feet/toes. Stand on your toes for a count of 10.

***

3.

Aerobic Exercises

Aerobic exercises include walking, skipping a rope, jogging (on a treadmill or in the park), cycling or spinning in the gym, swimming, aerobic classes in a gym, sports like tennis and basketball as well as everyday activities like climbing stairs, housework and gardening.

Swimming is a good option especially if you are overweight or obese because it does not put excessive pressure on the joints of the lower limbs.

To reap the most benefits from your aerobic exercise sessions, you should:

1. Exercise for at least 30 min each session

2. Reach your Target Heart Rate (THR) which is calculated by

220 - your age = maximum heart rate (MHR)

MHR x 0.65 = minimum target heart rate (MinTHR)

MHR x 0.80 = maximum target heart rate (MaxTHR)

For example, if you are 40 years old, 220 - 40 years = 180 your maximum heart rate (MHR)

180 (MHR) x 0.65 = 117 your minimum target heart rate (MinTHR)

180 (MHR) x 0.80 = 144 your maximum target heart rate (MaxTHR)

Therefore, as you exercise, you should ensure that your heart rate is between 117 and 144.

To know your heart rate per minute, take your pulse on your wrist or neck for one minute.

The following is a rough guide of target heart rates for different age groups:

If you are 20 years old, your Target Heart Rate (THR) per minute should be 130 - 160

If you are 30 years old, your Target Heart Rate (THR) per minute should be 123 – 152

If you are 40 years old, your Target Heart Rate (THR) per minute should be 117 – 144

If you are 50 years old, your Target Heart Rate (THR) per minute should be 110 – 136

If you are 60 years old, your Target Heart Rate (THR) per minute should be 104 – 128

If you are 70 years old, your Target Heart Rate (THR) per minute should be 97 – 120

If you are 80 years old, your Target Heart Rate (THR) per minute should be 91 – 112

Exercise Plan

You can modify this plan to suit your lifestyle and level of activity.

Exercise Activity for Week 1

Day 1

Whole body stretch to warm up

30 min walk at minimum THR

Whole body stretch to cool down

Day 2

Whole body stretch to warm up

10 push ups, 10 triceps dips, 10 crunches

Whole body stretch to cool down

Day 3

Whole body stretch to warm up

30 min walk at minimum THR

Whole body stretch to cool down

Day 4

Whole body stretch to warm up

10 squats, 10 lunges, 10 calf raises, 10 crunches

Whole body stretch to cool down

Day 5

Whole body stretch to warm up

30 min walk at minimum THR

Whole body stretch to cool down

Exercise Activity for week 2

Day 1

Whole body stretch to warm up

30 min walk/ jog at medium THR

Whole body stretch to cool down

Day 2

Whole body stretch to warm up

15 push ups, 15 bicep curls, 15 triceps dips, 15 crunches

Whole body stretch to cool down

Day 3

Whole body stretch to warm up

30 min walk/ jog at medium THR

Whole body stretch to cool down

Day 4

Whole body stretch to warm up

15 squats, 15 lunges, 15 calf raises, 15 crunches

Whole body stretch to cool down

Day 5

Whole body stretch to warm up

30 min walk/ jog at medium THR

Whole body stretch to cool down

Exercise Activity for week 3

Day 1

Whole body stretch to warm up

30 min walk/run maximum THR

Whole body stretch to cool down

Day 2

Whole body stretch to warm up

20 push ups, 20 bicep curls, 20 triceps dips, 20 crunches

Whole body stretch to cool down

Day 3

Whole body stretch to warm up

30 min walk/run maximum THR

Whole body stretch to cool down

Day 4

Whole body stretch to warm up

20 squats, 20 lunges, 20 calf raises, 20 crunches

Whole body stretch to cool down

Day 5

Whole body stretch to warm up

30 min walk/run maximum THR

Whole body stretch to cool down

Exercise Activity for week 4

Day 1

Whole body stretch to warm up

30 min walk/run maximum THR

Whole body stretch to cool down

Day 2

Whole body stretch to warm up

30 push ups, 30 bicep curls, 30 triceps dips, 30 crunches

Whole body stretch to cool down

Day 3

Whole body stretch to warm up

30 min walk/run maximum THR

Whole body stretch to cool down

Day 4

Whole body stretch to warm up

30 push ups, 30 bicep curls, 30 triceps dips, 30 crunches

Whole body stretch to cool down

Day 5

Whole body stretch to warm up

30 min walk/run maximum THR

Whole body stretch to cool down

* * * * *

8

STRESS MANAGEMENT PLAN

Learning and practicing relaxation techniques is a very effective way of managing stress. These relaxation techniques include:

1.

Meditation

Meditation is another effective relaxation technique for coping with stress. To meditate, simply lie down in a quiet place and take several deep breaths. Once your body begins to feel calmer, focus on your inhalation and on the pure oxygen entering your body. As you exhale, envision you whole body relaxing. You can also meditate on Scriptures like **With God all things are possible** (Matthew 19:26) and envisioning your stressful situation resolving miraculously.

***

2.

Abdominal Breathing

Abdominal breathing or deep breathing is one fastest ways of counteracting the body's stress response. It is done by inhaling through your nose until your abdomen rises, holding your breath for a few moments and then exhaling completely through your mouth until your abdomen collapses. This cycle of filling the lungs with air, pausing and then emptying them can be repeated for 15 minutes every day.

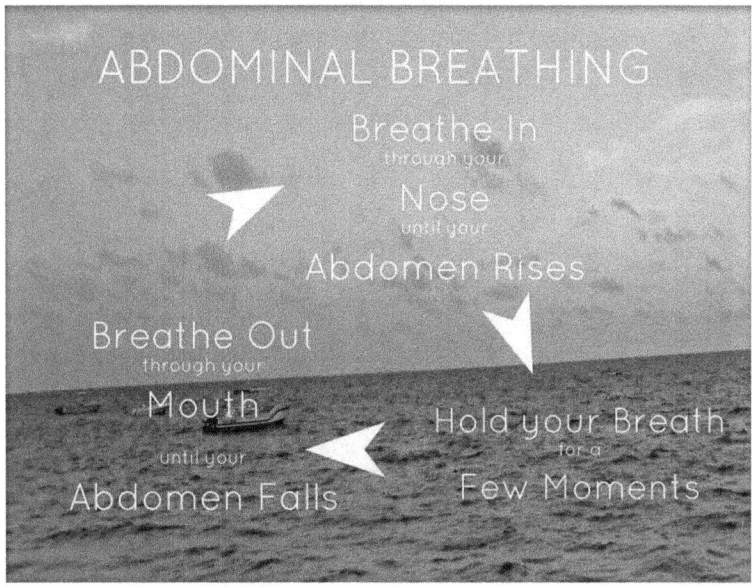

***

3.

Guided Imagery

Guided imagery is another effective relaxation technique. It involves visualizing yourself in a relaxing environment. Therefore close your eyes, take several deep breaths and use your mind's eye to see yourself relaxing on a beach or floating on a cloud or walking through a garden or whichever environment makes you feel relaxed. Use all your senses to immerse yourself in the restful environment by seeing soothing images, smelling appealing scents, hearing calming sounds, tasting and feeling your way through it. After you have enjoyed our visit, bring yourself gently back to reality.

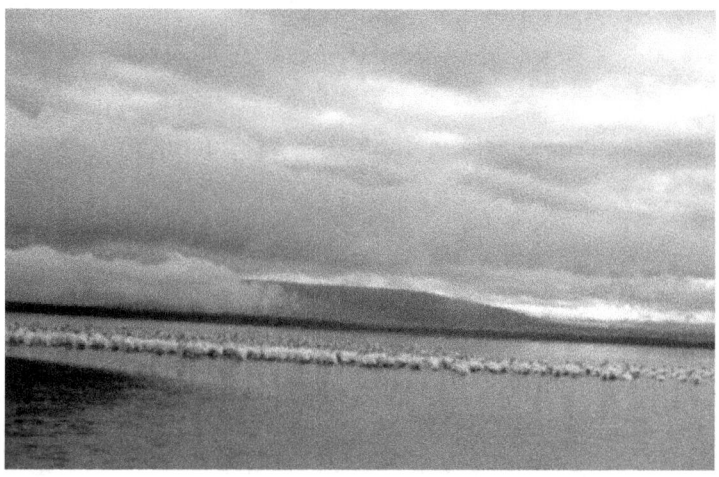

***

4.

Problem Solving Visualization

Visualization can also be used to manage stressful situations. To do this see yourself with your mind's eye in your most stressful situation and then envisioning yourself using various strategies to cope. For example you can imagine yourself dealing with a stressful boss by breathing deeply until you no longer feel distressed by their words or actions.

***

5.

Physical Exercise

When a person is stressed, they tense their muscles. Stretching exercises reduce this muscle tension and help a person feel relaxed.

Aerobic exercises help the body burn circulating stress hormones that contribute to the development of stress related illnesses.

Weight bearing exercises also aid in stress management since they demand concentration and help a person forget their problems.

Therefore engage in regular physical exercises to manage stress.

***

Relaxing Activities

Other relaxing activities that you can engage in to manage stress include:

1. Journaling since writing down uncensored feelings is a very effective method of catharsis. It is doubly effective when combined with writing lists of things you are thankful for.

2. Listening to calming music.

3. Engaging in hobbies that complement their main job

4. Helping less fortunate members of your society like visiting the sick in hospitals since this takes your mind off your problems

5. Drinking soothing herbal teas like chamomile and passionflower.

6. Eating foods which raise serotonin levels like turkey, salmon, chicken, cheese, chocolate, wholegrain bread.

7. Watching comedy since laughter relieves tension.

8. Spending time with your social support system.

***

Stress Management Plan

Stress Management Plan Week 1

Day 1

1. Abdominal breathing

2. Meditation

3. Physical Exercise

4. Watching Comedy

Day 2

1. Abdominal breathing

2. Meditation

3. Drinking herbal teas and eating serotonin rich foods

4. Watching Comedy

Day 3

1. Abdominal breathing

2. Meditation

3. Physical Exercise

4. Watching Comedy

Day 4

1. Abdominal breathing

2. Meditation

3. Drinking herbal teas and eating serotonin rich foods

4. Watching Comedy

Day 5

1. Abdominal breathing

2. Meditation

3. Physical Exercise

4. Watching Comedy

Day 6 and 7

1. Abdominal breathing 2. Meditation 3. Spending time with your social support system

Stress Management Plan Week 2

Day 1

1. Abdominal breathing

2. Guided imagery

3. Physical Exercise

4. Listening to Music

Day 2

1. Abdominal breathing

2. Guided imagery

3. Drinking herbal teas and eating serotonin rich foods

4. Listening to Music

Day 3

1. Abdominal breathing

2. Guided imagery

3. Physical Exercise

4. Listening to Music

Day 4

1. Abdominal breathing

2. Guided imagery

3. Drinking herbal teas and eating serotonin rich foods

4. Listening to Music

Day 5

1. Abdominal breathing

2. Guided imagery

3. Physical Exercise

4. Listening to Music

Day 6 and 7

1. Abdominal breathing 2. Guided imagery 3. Engaging in Complementary Hobbies

Stress Management Plan Week 3

Day 1

1. Abdominal breathing

2. Problem solving visualization

3. Physical Exercise

4. Journaling and writing gratitude lists

Day 2

1. Abdominal breathing

2. Problem solving visualization

3. Drinking herbal teas and eating serotonin rich foods

4. Journaling and writing gratitude lists

Day 3

1. Abdominal breathing

2. Problem Solving Visualization

3. Physical Exercise

4. Journaling and writing gratitude lists

Day 4

1. Abdominal breathing

2. Problem Solving Visualization

3. Drinking herbal teas and eating serotonin rich foods

4. Journaling and writing gratitude lists

Day 5

1. Abdominal breathing

2. Problem Solving Visualization

3. Physical Exercise

4. Journaling and writing gratitude lists

Day 6 and 7

1. Abdominal breathing 2. Problem Solving Visualization 3. Helping the less fortunate

Stress Management Plan Week 4

Day 1

1. Abdominal breathing

2. Meditation or Guided Imagery or Problem Solving Visualization (choose the one that has been most relaxing for you and practice it regularly)

3. Physical exercise

4. Watching Comedy or Listening to Music or Journaling and writing gratitude lists (choose the one that has been most relaxing for you and practice it regularly)

Day 2

1. Abdominal breathing

2. Meditation or Guided Imagery or Problem Solving Visualization (choose the one that has been most relaxing for you and practice it regularly)

3. Drinking herbal teas and eating serotonin rich foods

4. Watching Comedy or Listening to Music or Journaling and writing gratitude lists (choose the one that has been most relaxing for you and practice it regularly)

Day 3

1. Abdominal breathing

2. Meditation or Guided Imagery or Problem Solving Visualization (choose the one that has been most relaxing for you and practice it regularly)

3. Physical exercise

4. Watching Comedy or Listening to Music or Journaling and writing gratitude lists (choose the one that has been most relaxing for you and practice it regularly)

Day 4

1. Abdominal breathing

2. Meditation or Guided Imagery or Problem Solving Visualization (choose the one that has been most relaxing for you and practice it regularly)

3. Drinking herbal teas and eating serotonin rich foods

4. Watching Comedy or Listening to Music or Journaling and writing gratitude lists (choose the one that has been most relaxing for you and practice it regularly)

Day 5

1. Abdominal breathing

2. Meditation or Guided Imagery or Problem Solving Visualization (choose the one that has been most relaxing for you and practice it regularly)

3. Physical exercise

4. Watching Comedy or Listening to Music or Journaling and writing gratitude lists (choose the one that has been most relaxing for you and practice it regularly)

Day 6 and 7

1. Abdominal breathing

2. Meditation or Guided Imagery or Problem Solving Visualization (choose the one that has been most relaxing for you and practice it regularly)

3. Spending time with your social support system or Engaging in complementary hobbies or Helping the less fortunate (choose the one that has been most relaxing for you and practice it regularly)

###

ABOUT THE AUTHOR

Dr. Miriam Kinai is a medical doctor and freelance health writer/blogger.

You can visit her blog at http://www.MyBlogBookClub.com or follow her on twitter at http://twitter.com/AlmasiHealth

Email enquiries to almasihealthcare@yahoo.com with BOOKS as your subject.

*****

HERBS AND SPICES FOR THE COOK, HEALER AND BEAUTICIAN

Herbs and Spices for the Cook, Healer and Beautician uses color pictures and clear explanations to teach you about more than 70 healing herbs and spices.

You will learn about their:

* Therapeutic (healing) uses

* Drug interactions

* Contraindications (when not to use them)

* Cooking tips

* Beauty tips

*****

INTERNATIONAL GOURMET HERB AND SPICE BLENDS

International Gourmet Herb and Spice Blends teaches you how to prepare exotic herb and spice blends from around the world. You will discover the recipes for:

* Barbecue Rub, Cajun, Apple Pie and Pumpkin Pie Spice Mixes from America

* Pudding Spice Mix from Britain

* 5 Spice Mix from China

* Berbere Spice Mix from Ethiopia

* Curry Powder and Garam Masala from India

* Bouquet Garni, Herbs de Provence and Quatre Epices from France

* Herb Mix from Italy

* Jerk Seasoning from Jamaica

* Shichimi Togarashi from Japan

* Pilau Spice Blend from Kenya

* Chili Powder from Mexico

* Baharat Spice Blend from the Middle East

* Ras El Hanout from Morocco

*****

THE QUICK GOURMET CHEF

The Quick Gourmet is an essential culinary skills cookbook which teaches how to make simple, divine dishes.

You will learn how to make:

* Hot Chocolate Mixes and Drinks

* Hot Chai Tea Mixes and Drinks

* Hot Coffee Mixes and Drinks

* Sensational Smoothies

* Non-Dairy Smoothies

* Chocolate Covered Strawberries

* Chocolate Truffles

* Healthy Chicken Salads

* Healthy Tuna Salads

* Savory Salsas

* Herb Butter

* Cheese Dips and Sauces

* Gourmet Sandwiches

* Perfect Hard Boiled Eggs

* A Cheese Board

* Natural Food Color

*****

HOW TO STYLE AND PHOTOGRAPH FOOD

Regardless of whether you are an aspiring food blogger or you want to make money online selling stock photos, How To Style and Photograph Food, uses color pictures and clear explanations to teach you the food photography tips that can help you improve your digital camera photography skills so that you can begin photographing food like a pro.

You will learn:

* The equipment that you need

* How to set up the lighting

* How to prepare the stage

* How to style the food

* How to shoot the food

*****

HOW TO MAKE NATURAL SKIN CARE PRODUCTS VOLUME 1

How To Make Natural Skin Care Products Volume 1 by Dr Miriam Kinai is filled with recipes for making organic bath and body products for normal, sensitive, oily and dry skin types as well as therapeutic products to manage mature skin, prematurely aging skin, cellulite, eczema, psoriasis, ringworms, dandruff, thinning hair, menopausal symptoms, pre-menstrual tension (PMS), painful periods, arthritis, stress, sadness or depression, mental exhaustion and insomnia.

This book also teaches you the best vegetable oils, essential oils, natural butters and herbs to use when making products for different skin types physical conditions. You will learn how to make:

* Bath bombs

* Bath melts

* Bath salts

* Bath teas

* Body butters

* Body lotions

* Body scrubs

* Healing balms and body creams

* Herb infused oils

* Natural soap

How to Make Natural Skin Care Products Volume 1 will leave you with a clear understanding of how to make bath and beauty products to use in your home or to give as gifts or to sell and make money.

*****

ORGANIC SKIN CARE PRODUCT INGREDIENTS

Organic Skin Care Product Ingredients teaches you about the different natural substances that can be used to create natural bath and beauty products to use in your home or to give as gifts to your loved ones or to sell and make money.

You will learn about:

* Natural butters

* Natural clays

* Natural colorants

* Natural exfoliants

* Natural fragrances

* Natural oils

* Natural preservatives

*****

THE ESSENTIALS OF AROMATHERAPY ESSENTIAL OILS

The Essentials of Aromatherapy Essential Oils by Dr Miriam Kinai teaches you how to use aromatherapy oils to improve your physical, mental and emotional well being.

The author's experience as a medical doctor and clinical aromatherapy practitioner have enabled her to write a highly informative guide for those who want to utilize the healing benefits of these natural plant essences.

You will discover:

* The safety information and therapeutic uses of 18 essential oils

* How to blend essential oils

* The characteristics and uses of 14 carrier oils

* How to Dilute Essential Oils with Carrier Oils

* How to Use Essential Oils

* Cautionary Measures when using Essential Oils

* Numerous Essential Oil Recipes for bath products as well as skin care and hair care products

The Essentials of Aromatherapy Essential Oils will leave you with a clear understanding of how you can safely use aromatherapy essential oils to heal yourself naturally.

*****

CARRIER OILS GUIDE

Carrier Oils Guide teaches you the characteristics, health benefits and uses of commonly used carrier oils. You will learn about:

* Apricot Kernel Oil

* Avocado Oil

* Borage Seed Oil

* Calendula Oil

* Carrot Seed Oil

* Castor Oil

* Evening Primrose Oil

* Fractionated Coconut Oil

* Jojoba

* Olive Oil

* Rosehip Oil

* Sunflower Oil

* Sweet Almond Oil

* Virgin Coconut Oil

* Useful formulas for Diluting Essential Oils with Carrier Oils

*****

MEDICAL AROMATHERAPY FOR HEALTH PROFESSIONALS

Medical Aromatherapy for Healthcare Professionals by Dr Miriam Kinai teaches you how to use essential oils to treat physical diseases and emotional disorders.

The author's experience as a medical doctor and clinical aromatherapy practitioner have enabled her to write a highly informative guide for those who want to utilize the healing benefits of these natural plant essences.

You will discover how to use essential oils to:

* Treat skin diseases like acne, eczema and psoriasis

* Treat other physical diseases like high blood pressure, arthritis, coughs and colds

* Manage mental and emotional conditions like anxiety, depression, anger and stress

* Relieve the symptoms of menopause and premenstrual tension

* Lessen insomnia and impotence

Medical Aromatherapy for Healthcare Professionals is therefore an essential resource for holistic healthcare practitioners like massage therapists, naturopaths and herbalists.

It is also a useful resource for conventional medicine healthcare providers like physicians and nurses who want to begin practicing integrative medicine and for patients who want to improve their health naturally by using aromatherapy oils.

*****

AROMATHERAPY COURSE

Aromatherapy Course by Dr Miriam Kinai tutors you on how to use essential oils to improve your physical, mental and emotional well being.

The author's experience as a medical doctor and clinical aromatherapy practitioner have enabled her to create a highly informative course on how to use these natural plant essences.

You will learn:

* The safety information and therapeutic uses of essential oils like clary sage, eucalyptus, geranium, grapefruit, lavender, lemon, lemongrass, marjoram, orange (sweet), patchouli, peppermint, Roman chamomile, rose, rosemary, sandalwood, spearmint, tea tree and ylang ylang.

* The safety information and therapeutic uses of carrier oils like apricot kernel oil, avocado oil, borage seed oil, calendula oil, carrot seed oil, castor oil, evening primrose oil, fractionated coconut oil, jojoba, olive oil, rosehip oil, sunflower oil, sweet almond oil and virgin coconut oil.

* How to blend essential oils

* How to dilute essential oils with carrier oils

* How to administer essential oils

* How to make natural healing products from numerous aromatherapy recipes

* How to utilize the healing benefits of essentials oils even if you do not have prior training in aromatherapy

The Aromatherapy Course will leave you with a clear understanding of how you can heal yourself and your family naturally by using essentials oils on your body and in your home.

*****

DEALING WITH DEPRESSION NATURALLY

Dealing with Depression Naturally presents a holistic approach to managing depression with natural antidepressants. You will learn how to treat depression with:

* Aromatherapy

* Art therapy

* Christian Biblical principles

* Chromotherapy

* Diet therapy

* Eco-therapy

* Herbal therapy

* Home decor therapy

* Music therapy

* Phototherapy

* Exercise therapy

* Self-Psychotherapy

* Social therapy

* Talk therapy

* Vitamin therapy

* Writing therapy

*****

CHRISTIAN LIFE COACHING HANDBOOK

Christian Life Coaching Handbook offers a Biblical approach to managing different aspects of life.

You will learn:

* Christian anger management

* Christian conflict resolution

* Christian depression treatment

* Christian goal setting

* Christian marital stress management

* Christian stress management

* How to assert yourself

* How to defeat fear

* How to love yourself

* How to overcome shyness

* How to resist temptation

* How to stop being a people pleaser

*****

CHRISTIAN PERSONAL FINANCE

Christian Personal Finance teaches Biblical principles of money management.

You will learn:

* Christian financial stress management from people who were dealing with money stress like the Acts 3 beggar or credit issues like the widow in second Kings.

* Biblical prosperity principles from wealthy men and women of God like Isaac and the Proverbs 31 woman.

* Bible verses to use as spiritual warfare prayers and as Christian finance affirmations and Christian money meditations.

*****

ANTHOLOGY OF CHRISTIAN BIBLE SERMONS

Anthology of Christian Bible Sermons is a compilation of more than 20 Biblical rhema teachings which include:

* A New Christmas Message

* A New Easter Message

* Are You A Flamboyant Fig Tree Christian?

* Biblical Lessons for Purim from Queen Esther

* Can God Help Me If I Am Surrounded By Enemies?

* How Badly Do You Really Want It?

* Seed Words And The Powerful Tongue

* Spiritual AIDS

* The Three Levels Of Getting Lost

* Why Does God Allow Suffering?

* Your Life Is Your Ministry And Your Storm Is Your Message

* A Perfect God, Imperfect People, and Perfect Plans

* We Are Not Ignorant of His Devices

* How to Prepare for a Dangerous Journey

* Yes, God Can

* How to Serve the Body of Christ

* Conduits of God

* Go Back? Stand Still? Move Forward? Drown?

*****

CHRISTIAN SPIRITUAL WARFARE

Christian Spiritual Warfare teaches you the awesome Bible verses you can use as spiritual warfare prayers, Christian affirmations and in your Christian meditation sessions as you fight your spiritual battles.

You will learn how to fight for the following with Bible verses:

* Marriage * Children * Health

* Christian Faith * Christian Ministry

* Country

* Finances * Job * Business

* Peace of Mind * Restoration * Self Esteem * Self Love

You will also learn how to fight against the following with Bible verses:

* Addiction * Temptation

* Being Single * Infertility

* Opposition * Oppression

* Worry * Fear

* Feelings of Condemnation * Confusion

* Danger * Death * Despair * Discouragement

* Impatience * Insomnia * Laziness * Loneliness

* Poverty * Pride * Sadness

* Vengeance * Weakness

* A Foul Mouth * Lying

*****

DARK SKIN DERMATOLOGY COLOR ATLAS

Dark Skin Dermatology Color Atlas is filled with clear explanations and color photos of skin, hair, and nail diseases affecting people with skin of color or Fitzpatrick skin types IV, V, and VI.

Topics covered include Acne Vulgaris, Alopecia Areata, Anal Warts, Angioedema, Aphthous Ulcers, Atopic Dermatitis, Blastomycosis, Blister Beetle Dermatitis or Nairobi Fly Dermatitis, Cellulitis, Chronic Ulcers, Confetti Hypopigmentation, Cutaneous T Cell Lymphoma, Cutaneous Tuberculosis, Dermatitis Artefacta, Erythema Nodosum,

Exfoliative Erythroderma, Gianotti Crosti Syndrome, Hand Dermatitis, Hemangioma, Herpes Zoster, Ichthyosis, Ingrown Toenails, Irritant Contact Dermatitis, Kaposi Sarcoma, Keloids, Keratoderma Blenorrhagica, Klippel Trenaunay Weber Syndrome, Leishmaniasis, Leprosy, Leukonychia, Lichen Nitidus, Lichen Planus,

Lichenoid Drug Eruption, Linear Epidermal Nevus, Linear IgA Dermatosis (LAD), Lipodermatosclerosis, Lymphangioma Circumscriptum, Miliaria, Molluscum Contagiosum, Neurofibromatosis, Nickel Dermatitis, Onychomadesis, Onychomycosis, Palmoplantar Eccrine Hidradenitis, Papular Pruritic Eruption (PPE), Paronychia, Pellagra, Pemphigus Foliaceous,

Pemphigus Vulgaris, Piebaldism, Pityriasis Rosea, Pityriasis Rubra Pilaris, Plantar Hyperkeratosis, Plantar Warts, Poikiloderma, Postinflammatory Hyperpigmentation and Hypopigmentation, Post Topical Steroids Hypopigmentation, Psoriasis, Pyogenic Granuloma or Lobular Capillary Hemangioma, Scabies, Seborrheic Dermatitis, Steven Johnson Syndrome (SJS) and Toxic Epidermal Necrolysis (TEN),

Sunburn, Systemic Sclerosis, Tinea Capitis, Tinea Pedis, Tinea Versicolor, Traction Alopecia, Urticaria, Vasculitis, Vitiligo, and Xanthelasma.

*****

www.ingramcontent.com/pod-product-compliance
Lightning Source LLC
Chambersburg PA
CBHW070554290526
45790CB00002B/677